A Special Vow

To care for and love forever

Michael A. Zuniga

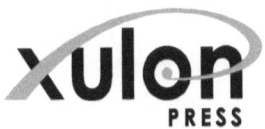

xulon PRESS

Acknowledgements

I would like to thank Mike Valentino, my editor, who felt strongly about my story and the beautiful way he transformed my feelings into words. Jean would have loved that. She loved to learn new words and couldn't wait to use them.

My daughter Theresa Huether and my son Frank Zuniga for their love and support in my volunteering ministry for my church (Sacred Heart Church). I thank two very special ladies who worked with me for 16 years, Bev Courtney and Myrna Rose who kept my spirit up as we visited the patients at Turlock Nursing. This was the facility where I placed Jean. I would take Jean every Tuesday morning in her wheelchair for 16 months and she loved to visit the patients. We did this right to the last week and her smile was a blessing to all. I especially want to thank Xulon Press for their patience when I found it difficult to finish the manuscript. They understood my feelings and when Jean passed away on February 16, 2009, I felt free to focus on my book. I did not plan it but I finished the last page on 8-12-2009 the same day we planned our original wedding date 8-12-1950.

Thank you, Lord, for the beautiful years you gave to us. And thanks to all the people who helped me when I needed their support.

Introduction

When I stood at the foot of the Altar and placed the wedding ring on her finger and spoke my wedding vows, I had no idea how special they were until I heard our doctor tell me that my precious wife had started to show the early signs of Alzheimer's disease. This was in 2004 and we had been married 54 years and still very much in love and full of plans. Our family was starting to get larger with the great grandchildren coming along and more good things to come. We were stunned to put it mildly when we were told that Jean has this disease that cannot be cured and in time Jean will have no memory of what we held dear.

My first thought was why did this happen to Jean. My Jean who always made time to help people. She was my silent partner. I did the talking and she did the listening. She made the time to listen. When she finally did have something to say it was always the right thing to do. I learned so much from her. She always said we had a special kind of love. I chose her to be my wife for the rest of my life and to this date I love her more than I did on that special day when I spoke with my heart to love and to cherish until death do we part.

This is our love story and if in time of trouble it helps you to stay together and with the help of our Lord and Savior Jesus Christ you too will share a special kind of love.

Chapter One

Meeting Jean and our Courtship

J ean and I were born and raised in San Francisco. We attended Catholic schools and pretty much grew up in the same type of neighborhoods and did a lot of the same things. We enjoyed being around people and got into projects that would help others. Some would call that being a volunteer. Whatever it was we loved it and that was what made us work so well together.

We both dated and had good friends to hang around with and keep us busy. Jean started to work full time after high school and joined a club of young adults called Young Christian Workers. Their purpose was to get together every week to find new friends with the same goals. They had Bible studies and discussions on finding jobs and also how to plan for a good Christian future.

They had many activities like weekly dances and lots of outings. My four sisters also joined and met Jean before I did. Since they liked her, they mentioned how nice it would be if we could meet and become friends.

This came later when I went to a party with my best friend. There was Jean as cute as a little bug's ear. We had a good time and my best friend managed to talk her into taking her home. I had the car but he had the girl so she became his girl and like a good friend I stepped aside — but gosh she was so cute.

Time went by and one day my best friend asked me to get a date and go to a special dance with him and his new girlfriend. I had trouble getting a date so he suggested that I ask Jean, who he never dated, or even spoke about since we met her at that party and I drove her to her home. I always had her on my mind. I couldn't believe this was happening and so I jumped at the chance to call on Jean at her work. She worked at the Emporium Department store in downtown San Francisco. She was thrilled to see me and agreed to go with me, and of course she knew my sisters so it was OK to accept a short notice date.

We both knew there was something special about our meeting. Our good times were the beginning of Mike and Jean always together.

We couldn't stop talking about all the things we liked and wanted to do. I could talk forever about how much we were alike and just being together was so wonderful.

I took her home and started to meet her family and there again we all felt like one big happy family.

When I asked her if I could see her again soon we both laughed at the thought of making it the next day and so it went. We were dating on a daily basis. I would pick her up after work and we could spend hours just talking away about nothing important. Just sharing and feeling good just being together.

Sometimes I would drop by during my lunch break and see her working at the information booth where all kinds of people asked her questions about what to do in San Francisco, or leave messages with her to relay to others.

This was long before the day of cell phones. People called her by her first name and it was like a little village store instead of downtown big city.

My family really loved her at first sight. Even my father called her "my Jean."

Her side of the family was also pleased to see her so happy.

Her dad had died when she was four and her mother had to raise five kids all by herself. Jean was 18 when her mother was confined to a hospital with diabetes and tuberculosis and not given any chance to live. We visited her on Sundays and I knew how happy she was to see her little baby being taken in by a large family who loved her.

She lived long enough for me to ask her for her blessing in marrying her daughter. A grand lady, Jean learned from her how to raise a family without complaining. I myself experienced Jean's forgiving nature and I give her full credit for all the things we did to complete 57 years of marriage.

Jean did not really have a family house. When her mother passed away all her sisters and two brothers were adults over 18 and so they lived apart. Jean was thrilled to have our place to call home.

We had a five-bedroom flat, which was built like a huge boarding house. It was three stories high and three of my aunts lived in the flat above ours. I want to explain that a flat was just like an apartment except that it had its own front door leading to the street.

Jean's uncle was a Franciscan priest and he helped by bringing groceries to Jean's place and was available to provide some sort of parental influence.

When he passed away he asked his friend who was also a Franciscan priest to take over and watch over the family, especially the girls.

He placed Jean and her sister in an apartment for young ladies and that was what Jean called home. She was really close to where she worked so she could walk to work, and the church where we got married was right around the corner.

The young Christian Workers Club was next to the church so her whole world was in a tight little corner.

By now I joined the club so I was seeing a lot of Jean and every day was like heaven on earth. Everyone knew someday we would be married and it was in 1949 that I asked her to marry me. I gave her the engagement ring on Christmas Eve that year and we began to make serious plans for our future.

Our courtship was so special. The people at my work met Jean and the wedding showers were a lot of fun for Jean. I was already a fixture at her workplace because I was there every day.

We knew we were young to get married but our love was strong and we just knew God was with us every step of the way.

The date was set for August 12, 1950 and we enjoyed being together. The problem we had was ending the day and being unable to say goodnight. I don't know how we managed to do our work with so little sleep. We would agree to not see each other for one night but sure enough we ended phoning up each other and talking ourselves into getting together for just a few minutes. It all sounded good until we met and next thing we just couldn't say goodnight.

God took care of everything and even though we did not have a personal relationship with Him we always were aware of His presence in our lives and we prayed to Him and went to church often. Also the club focused on getting to know more about God so we thanked Him for what He was doing in our lives.

Jean's priest/guardian Father Aidan, was a tremendous source of spiritual strength and we could go to him when we needed some advice. Of course at 21 we thought we knew it all.

Father Aidan was a wise priest and he would only smile when we tried to supply the answer to a tough question.

Later on as we grew old we'd see the young people struggling to find the solution to a good marriage and we just could not convince them to just let go and let God do the work in their lives.

I just can't thank God enough for His patience with me and for the patience Jean had to cope with a strong willed person like myself.

Our kids saw that in us and I am sure as they get older they will also get stronger in love and give everything to God. Oh to have the wisdom of an 80 year old and the youth of a twenty year old. Jesus knows the answer to this mystery and all I could say is to trust in God and listen for His voice.

We were doing our best and I am sure we had a lot of people praying for us and wishing us well.

The girls at the Emporium gave us a super treat as a surprise gift. We went to dinner at the Fairmont Hotel which was a pretty pricey place and after dinner when we asked for the bill we were told that the Emporium had paid the bill as a special wedding gift to us.

The San Francisco Chronicle wrote the story and like I said before San Francisco was a large city but in a certain way it became a little village.

We both felt so blessed and could not believe all the good things that we were experiencing.

Then the unexpected thing happened. I had joined the Marine Corps reserve in 1947 to delay my being drafted as I was planning to attend college. I changed my mind about college after a year but stayed active in the reserves because it was fun and never thought I would regret doing that.

I mentioned before the wedding date was set for August 12, 1950. All the wedding invitations were ready to be mailed and everything was set to go. There was nothing left to do just show up for the wedding.

That's what I thought except that I received a phone call from a friend of mine who told me that our reserve unit had been activated and we were supposed to report for active duty at any moment. I thought it was a joke. I could not believe what I heard but it didn't matter. I was going to call and get myself excused. I had completed my time of three years and I had it written in my contract that I would only be called in if we were in a war.

I sure found out how wrong I was. My commanding officer told me that I would be called real soon and I better report or they will come after me even if they had to go to the wedding to get me. I was told it was a police action because North Korea had invaded South Korea and we were going to the defense of the South.

I said where is Korea and why don't they have a police force. Also my time had been extended another year so here I was helpless and sure enough I received my official notice to report to my base and I was stunned.

Jean could not believe what had happened and neither could everyone else. Our country sure gets into wars in the strangest way. I called someone with authority but in a very sweet way I was told that I would be breaking the law if I refused to report. So here I am saying to Jean, "I'm sorry, Hon, you have to cancel everything so I can go overseas to take care of some kind of police action."

Even my boss tried to get me off.

Next thing you know I get the official notice that we will be shipping out as soon as possible.

We decided to wait till I got back because there was no way we could have the wedding and most important there was no way the government would support Jean while I was in the service. No provision was in effect to take care of wives unless it was a war and then Congress would pass a bill giving family support. How is that for a new way to make it hard to serve your country.

There is the right way and then there is the Marine way. They call that Semper Fi.

I reported for duty and Jean came down to Los Angeles to say good bye and it was so sad to see her board the bus and knowing she would be all alone till I got back. I will never forget that day. We were so close to becoming man and wife and here I was going overseas to a country I never heard of and was not convinced that I was needed to solve their problems.

This was a real challenge and again I had to trust our Lord more than ever before. I just knew He should be in charge of my life but it was so easy to just say forget it and go at it all by myself. I thought of my Jean praying by herself in some church and that made me feel like I owed it to her to tough it out and return to her as soon as possible.

Chapter Two

Military Life Away from Jean

Our good Lord calmed us down after we ran around trying to find the right thing to do. We could have gone to Reno for a quick wedding but that would not have solved the problem of how Jean was to live till I returned. We both felt deep in our hearts that we should wait and just trust that God would see us through all this. I know our hearts were broken but we gave strength to each other and we felt more in love than ever before so that was it and we started to look ahead to the future.

Here I was a brand new United States Marine. I never received basic training. I was classified as an airplane mechanic and that was the only training I received. We attended two week-ends a month at the Alameda Naval Air Station just across the Bay. We learned how to repair airplanes how to park them and get them ready for action as fast as we could. Down time was important so practice and more practice made our day.

However, when we reported for duty we were changed to Rifleman and we were to be prepared to be part of a large invasion force to land in Korea in September. Keep in mind that we were called in June and reported in August to ship out in September. This may seem like a lot of time but remember, three months ago I was sitting in a desk doing my job and looking ahead to a beautiful wedding with my lovely bride planning our future together. No one knew what to do with us after we were activated. We were not at war and we were asked to die for our country. Thirty-five thousand did within three years and many wounded not just from enemy fire but from frostbite caused from a frigid winter that sometimes dropped to 38 degrees below zero. The fact was we had clothing handed down from World War II and it was for warm weather. It took a while before we got the cold weather clothing and snow boots were so welcomed. We also had so many bankruptcies, broken marriages, and loss of businesses because some men did not have enough time to settle up their civilian affairs. We were being rushed and now they did not know what to do with us. This is why we did the right thing. At one time we were told that we were not going to go overseas and then that was changed.

We finally were told of our shipping out day and Jean came down to say good-bye. We went to a theater and kissed and hugged all through the movie. We never saw the movie but we held on to each other with all the love we had for each other. I returned to the base hurting from all that was happening. I prayed to the Lord to take care of Jean and my life was in His hands.

Korea was called the Forgotten War and I could see why. The whole thing was a mess from the beginning so it took awhile before we got squared away and then it was like after Pearl Harbor, we became a smooth running machine.

The day came September 1, 1950, and we were stuffed into trucks headed to the ship and we all felt like we were saying good-bye to everything we held dear. The worst feeling was when we were all standing at the rail of the ship looking at the coast as it started to fade away in the distance and then it finally disappeared from sight. I couldn't hold back tears and I was not alone. The feeling is hard to describe but it was like the beginning of the end and that I was not coming back.

I was so glad to hear a booming voice over the loudspeaker shout, "Now hear this, all men report to your station for evacuation drill," and that brought us down to earth and my military life overseas began.

I had never been on a ship this far away from shore. I heard the Pacific Ocean was called the Blue Pacific and now I know why. The sight of it was magnificent and with the blue sky to match, it took your breath away. Then at night the endless sky was full of stars which seemed to touch the ocean. Only God could have created that scene. I heard that old time sailors used the stars to guide them from one place to another. God was showing off for us and that sight made my day.

When we went below it was another story. Three decks down it smelled like diesel oil. This transport was a converted luxury liner ship named the USS Norton. They sure did a good job in converting it because you could not tell it was a luxury liner and that people had ever paid to sail on it. It served its purpose in loading up with the maximum amount of troops to transport. When I went to sleep I felt I was sleeping on the wall and in fact I really was. The bunks were secured to the sides of the ship five high. They folded down like shelves. You could not sit up once you climbed into your bunk. Once in awhile in your sleep you could want to sit up and you could really hurt your head as it scraped on the above bunk.

The next day everyone woke up to a bad day. The ship's motion was up and down and then it would sort of roll side to side, perfect to get you seasick. It was hard to go to the mess hall and try to eat. The dishes and cups kept moving away from you and then they would come back. Then someone told us that September was hurricane season. That was all we needed to hear.

After a few days we started to get used to this. The food stayed in our stomachs and we were getting our sea legs so we could walk around without reaching for the handrails to keep from falling down.

Every night we had a beautiful prayer service, which everyone attended. We sang some hymns and listened to the Word proclaimed. The stars shined extra bright and you could feel angels all around and the presence of the Lord was for sure.

We started to make new friends and it was good to share our lives with one another. We could complain and let our anger get out and get rid of our frustrations. Also it was good to know that we were not alone in our feelings.

We knew we had a job to do and it bonded us to each other and we became good friends willing to do anything for each other.

We all worried about what would happen if we never returned and who would take care of our loved ones. Our chaplain talked about all this at our prayer service and told us to give it all to God.

The ones who did not know God started asking guys like me to tell them all about praying to God and would He take them back if they went back to going to church. This led to interesting conversations and sometimes late at night some one would stand by my bunk and just talk about God and ask me some real good questions.

The next day I would hear someone say how it was just like going to church to hear us talk. It made me feel good to know the Lord was using me to talk to others to know Him better. The uncertainty of all things to happen did make people aware of the need to have God become more a part of our lives.

This was a long trip and living in such a crowd you got to know everyone. We waited in line everywhere we went and that part was tough to take

We attended sessions where they taught us the tactics of war. How to shoot weapons we had and what to do when we were engaged in battle. I could tell that I was not going to be working on airplanes in the near future. We were told to think of our enemy as a thing and not as a person so that when the time came to shoot him we would not have any problem. I had never thought of killing anyone ever and in fact I had trouble going fishing and seeing a fish die because I took him out of water. The country boys loved to hear that story and they would tell me how they hunted with their fathers when they were only four years old. Good for them. I just felt life was special and I did not enjoy someone else's life style. Then someone would tell me that it was better to take their life instead of them taking mine so shoot first. Our chaplain tried to paint a better picture and told us of the good we were doing by protecting the South Koreans from being invaded. He also reminded us how David defeated the enemy because he had God on his side.

We were being molded into a mean fighting machine in only ten days. When we were firing at moving targets I kept on thinking of being part of the invasion force and that kept me from getting a good night's sleep. Of course the smell of oil and the ship rolling back and forth also helped keeping us from sleeping well.

I was writing letters to Jean every day like a diary and I knew Jean was doing the same. Once we were at a place where we could mail them we knew we would be in touch and that would be real special.

We were getting closer to our destination and sure enough we heard that we were going to be a big part of an invasion on the east coast of Korea. We were going to be in the third wave. I asked what is a wave? I was told we were the third group of people to try and land on the beach. I always loved the beach and back home I would love to run into the water and dive under the waves and come shooting up full of energy and kept doing that again and again. Now I am also being told that it was similar to that except we would have our clothes on with 60 pounds of equipment on us and when we land we shoot people waiting for us and trying to keep us from landing on their beach. I saw this in movies with John Wayne but this time I was in it and I could get killed. Some old vet told me not to worry because if it's my turn to go I may never feel a thing. How comforting is that?

Like I said the Lord was good to me. We soon found out that because we were too slow in getting to Korea some other outfit would take our place and we would be headed to Japan and wait for a new assignment. That was a miracle and I knew prayers were being answered. When Jean's mail came I read how many times she was going to confession and praying for me. I could just see God smiling at her and telling her not to worry because He was taking care of me. I thanked Him for being the faithful God that He is and prayed for more grace to really know Him more.

We finally docked in Japan and began to plan another invasion on the east coast of Korea.

We heard about the invasion we missed out on and it was not pretty but our troops landed and were heading north so we knew we had to hurry and do our part to complete the task.

When we arrived at our base there was a ton of mail for me and that was all I needed to pick me up and give me new life. She was full of news and I got caught up on all the family news. Our home news-paper had written an article on how we had to postpone our wedding and we were going to be married as soon as I came back home.

I was the envy of my group and they even asked me if I was paying someone to write to me. They knew everyone knew Jean and I shared that special kind of love.

I had a real buddy by the name of Axel Rosengren from St. Paul, Minnesota. He worked in the supply warehouse and his office was our nightly meeting place for the two of us to get together and write our letters to our loved ones. He was married and his wife was to have a baby around November and he was so sad knowing that he was going to miss the birth. We had a lot to share because we both became Marines and called up in the same way.

We became great friends and it was fun to see both wives writing daily and both of us sending them mail as well.

We had a lot to share and we could pick our selves up when we were down instead of hitting the road and going after every lady of the night near our base and surrender to their offers of, "Marine, do you want to have a good time?"

We took one day at a time and did the best we could.

The time came for our next invasion. Here we go again with the wave thing and again we are the third wave so again I worry. This time they tell us to go light on our ammunition and as soon as we are on the beach ammo carriers will re-supply us and go from there. I wonder what happens if I need to fire up a lot of bullets and run out before I get more?

Jean always said I worried too much. I agreed and told her to teach me her secret. Of course I knew. Jesus always took care of my Jean.

Ready or not here we come! We boarded landing barges. These huge boats opened in front and we waded into the water and headed to shore. They were so round at the bottom that at times we thought they would roll over. Worry, worry, worry.

I did not know the Sea of Japan was so big. It was like another ocean. We finally made it to our destination and we were ready to go. Then the second miracle happened. Yes, the invasion was held up because the bay was heavily mined and the Navy could not clear the water of special Russian made mines that were timed to explode at different times. That meant it would take several runs to detonate each mine. We were told to stay nearby and wait. Our ship along with the others anchored off shore. We felt relieved and I of course thanked the Lord for another special intervention. Then while we were starting to get bored we heard the sound of a helicopter and it was our mail coming out to our ships.

Jean's love poured out of the envelopes and I could smell her as I kissed her handwriting. I missed her so much and I felt bad for those guys who stopped getting any mail.

They enjoyed seeing me reading my mail and I sure shared the cookies Jean would send me along with the sport pages so we kept up with our home teams.

After a few days we officially called off the so-called invasion because the South Korean armed forces had run up the entire peninsula and had the North Koreans in full retreat.

We unloaded and set up camp in the port city of Wonsan.

What a difference it was. Here I was marching into Wonsan like a conquering hero and I was worried about surviving the invasion with lots of casualties. I thanked God for all that was happening because he sure took care of us. We seem to be aware of the big things he does but just surviving a single day we could and should thank Him for that but we take it for granted and give ourselves all the credit.

Once we set up the airstrip near the hotel our planes started coming in and we were assigned the duty of perimeter guard. We would be on duty four hours on and four hours off. The hotel looked cozy but it was like a huge icebox. All the windows were broken out and covered with plywood. Each room had a metal box where we would burn wood or anything that could be burned to produce heat so we could stay warm in the bitter cold as well as heat our canned rations. We built a mess hall, which was nice but if we went to eat and wait in line we found the only difference in eating out was that it was the same food except they would use larger cans. We ate when we could in our rooms and didn't have to wait in line. The weather was always 40 below zero so it was no picnic to go up in the hills and climb into a foxhole. We could not light a fire to keep warm because the enemy was looking for that. After we finished our four hours we returned and climbed into our sleeping bags and just as I began to feel warm someone would yell, "Next unit for duty, wake up." I could swear it was only one-hour sleep. After awhile we started to look half-dead. The good part was when our mail came and there was Jean warming me up with her love and I could hear her sweet voice as I read every word. God was so good in giving me that beautiful angel right out of Heaven for my very own. Her news was only good news. She wrote about everything and I could picture in my mind the places she went to and all my family taking real good care of her and her friends keeping her busy and making sure she had plenty of company.

The time came that we had to move up further north as our First Marine Division pushed up and we had to give them major support. Each time I packed I noticed my mail was taking up more room. Some guys burned their mail but I just couldn't do that so I just kept them in my backpack and had less clothes than I should have.

We seldom changed clothes anyway and we smelled anyway so who cared. Try taking a cold shower or just taking off your clothes in minus 40-degree weather. Growing beards was the norm and definitely no haircuts. What a sight we were.

I wrote to Jean and told her we might be home for Christmas because we were getting closer to the Chinese border and it looked like the end of this so-called Police Action. How wrong I was! We should never believe all that we hear. China was a little nervous about our troops getting too close to their borders so they put pressure on our government and to avoid conflict with China they agreed to stop and return to the place we started from and renegotiate territorial boundaries. We could not imagine giving up all we gained at the expense of 45,000 lost soldiers and all we were going through which no one seemed to care much about. Our attitude was sorry we came, thanks for the invitation and please call us the next time you need a policeman.

The orders were passed down RETREAT! Well, it sounded right except China did not wait for troop withdrawal, they attacked with hundreds of thousands of so-called volunteers. The Marines were the last of our troops to get the orders, so we found ourselves surrounded from all sides and China was going to wipe out our entire division and make sure the whole world would be totally impressed with their power. How wrong they were! We fought out of that trap and with our Navy helping us by support fire from their big gunships in the harbor. We boarded the ships and headed south to safety and a huge tactical defeat for our side. I was so tired from all we went through and with hardly no sleep I remember sitting near the docks and shellfire going over our heads and I was writing some notes to myself to put in my next letter. I wrote to Jean, I hope we can get out but I can now say for sure we won't be home for Christmas. Then I could remember my thinking of the shepherds in the fields watching their flock and seeing the star announcing the birth of Christ. You betcha we are going to make it and God the Father is getting us out of here.

Pusan Harbor was way down south and that was where we were headed. No more shooting and the sun was shining. It was like coming from Alaska to California. We marched into town where people lined up on the street to greet us because they had heard we had no chance of getting out with the Chinese army boasting how they were going to destroy us. Here we were a smelly bunch and ugly looking too but proud Marines and I was proud of what we accomplished.

At our base, after cleaning up (and that was quite a job) I heard the most beautiful words in the whole world "MAIL Call." I read every letter over and over just to absorb all the love Jean poured into each word. She worried about not hearing from me and seeing the newspaper articles about all our problems. She was hoping for any news from me. I had just mailed my bundle and it would be several days before she would know I was okay.

We are now considered stand-by troops and in the meantime because we were out of the danger zone we were re-classified Air Plane Mechanics. We got back to working on airplanes and sleeping in beds. Also the food was much better and once in a while we had food cooked in the kitchen. We soon got orders to go back to Japan and it was to be our permanent assignment. The new base was at Itami Air Base. When we asked where it was, we were told it's in the town of Itami just south of Osaka, of course. Jean would be happy I was in Japan. I think we were sent there to make us feel better after all we went through. I felt better about the whole thing. I was able to think more clearly about our future and I felt the worst was behind me. I started finding more space to put my letters away instead of carrying them in my back pack. I could not believe I had six months of her letters and she had the same from me. I did a lot of witnessing about God's love and being loyal to our loved ones back home. Our mail told our story and love needs no language. I remember Jean always telling me to listen to her heart because she could never say the right thing and I now knew what she meant. Jean prayed and prayed and her trips to the church gave me so much strength.

When I read the last word my eyes were moist but I didn't care. All I knew was that she loved me and Our dear Lord just got me through pure Hell. I will praise Him and thank Him forever. All I needed was a memory eraser to forget that all we did was for naught. We were back where we started and headed to Itami Air Base. We had done a great job and Japan was happy to have us back. There was a good feeling knowing that we were not hated for the Atom bomb thing. The towns were clean and busy with lots of happy people selling their wares. Our planes started coming in and we got them ready in quick time so they could return to their carriers and join the fighting. The neutral zone was the 38th parallel but the fighting was still going on to secure strategic positions and so men were still being killed but now it was being called a war. Years later after the battles ceased it was called the Forgotten War. A lot of people sure wanted to forget this war. Anyway, here we were in our new home and counting the days we would return to our real home. We were kept busy and the time went fast and before you know it we had been over seas for one year. Rumors were flying that we would be home by year's end. I said I would never believe rumors again but this was too good to keep from Jean. I told her that the troops were being rotated with fresh troops coming from the States and to start planning for our wedding in six months. This sounded premature but what it did was keep us focused on our wedding and that would keep our morale up. By September we really started to hear more and more about our replacements so I felt so good and I know Jean started some serious planning. It wasn't long before we were assured that we would be leaving Japan in December and we would be in San Francisco by Christmas. It was a long summer and not much happened except I was promoted to sergeant and boy did they ever try to recruit me for another year. I said no thank you I have a green eyed angel waiting for me and I plan to spend the rest of my life with her. Military life could be sweet but too many wars happen and memories of war were not too good. I was blessed with great friends to keep my spirit up and it was hard to keep focused on the present when all I could think of was getting home. The time came when we were officially on the list to go home and I know Jean must have jumped with joy when I told her to set up the date for the 12th of January if it was okay with her. All was set and now we could count the day and we could hear the minutes tick away.

Before we boarded the ship Jean sent me a copy of our newspaper and they had written up the story of our homecoming and mentioned how Jean and her Marine were going to be married after waiting two years since we postponed the wedding in 1950. We were a big story and I was proud to be a part of it. I felt like I could swim faster than the ship and it was the longest 10 days of my life until finally we spotted the lights on the Golden Gate Bridge. Everyone went nuts! Cheering the sights and arriving at night the city all lit up was a sight to behold. All was great except that we were told we had to wait for the morning before we docked so the newspaper people could film us coming into port and for the whole world to see us arrive. Then I was told that nobody was getting off because the ship would leave for San Diego. I was shocked and of course I went to our chaplain and after explaining my situation he gave me permission to leave with orders to report to camp in San Diego before the troops arrived.

I agreed and when we docked I remember seeing Jean waving her hands and I ran into her arms. We kissed hugged and screamed with joy and I am sure bells in Heaven rang. I had a great day with all my family and made sure to set things up to take a plane to San Diego. I started to question why God made such a problem for me but I should have known better. When God does things He does things big. By arriving on my own I was registered with a group of World War II veterans headed for immediate discharge. The reserves from my ship were to remain on active service for another six months. I phoned Jean from San Diego and told her I was discharged and heading home for good.

I arrived Christmas Eve and home to stay. God is so good and I was learning to trust Him more. We want everything now and can't get enough so this tells me just how patient God is with each one of us. I know now I didn't thank Him enough. Here He is handing me an immediate discharge and all I could think of was how I had to catch a plane to San Diego and yes I am truly sorry for offending my God with such ungratefulness. All my friends on the ship were processed and sent to another base for at least six more months. They were disappointed because they too thought they would get out. They were shocked to learn that I was released and went home to stay.

A very happy ending to my military career.

Chapter Three

Our Wedding, Honeymoon and Starting our Family

I was so happy to finally come home and not worry about catching a plane or leaving Jean for any length of time. We just held hands and loved every minute of being as close together as we could and wanted to be alone but it was impossible to get away when so much of my family wanted to share every moment with us. My company phoned me at home to tell me that my job was waiting for me and to hurry up. Then personal friends also called to get together. The newspaper did a good job of reporting our arrival. They wrote about the Marine reserves who were rushed to war and all the hardships that we had to endure. Then of course they mentioned our story and you know how people love an under dog story. The whole list of names from our ship was printed so all my friends had no trouble finding my name. Like the Z word for Zuniga the last name on the list. I knew that with God's help I was the first off the ship.

It took awhile to get used to my old life. Jean and I had lots of time to catch up on what was new. I don't know how she did it but she had arranged everything so that we didn't have much to do. The wedding plans were just like we had set them up and it felt like I never had left. Those two years were so hard on us but again we can thank God for all He did for us. Our love was tested by fire and we just knew all was meant to be.

The day came, January 12, 1952. Everyone was there. The people from my work, Jean's store and all our friends from the club and family relatives and friends. Jean was a living doll.

As she came down that long aisle with her long chestnut brown hair and green eyes I wanted to run away with her right then. I waited enough for her but then I realized that this was only the beginning. We had our whole life together and if you ever felt peace this was the time to have and to care for the rest of my life.

Jean did a wonderful job and the whole service was so beautiful. It made me forget how I felt when I had to leave her two summers ago and I just couldn't see that far ahead. Prayer and trusting God does help. I need God to teach me His way still. I worried that maybe some Marine official would be sending me a letter ordering me to get back to duty because they found out I was released too early. Jean was right - I worry too much.

The reception was like an old-fashioned picnic in the park. Nothing was catered. Food was cooked at home of friends and family. Plenty of joy all around and I am sure bells were ringing in heaven and I could see Jean's uncle-priest leading the parade The time came to depart and at last we were headed for that life that we thought we were never to have. My loving Jean was mine and I was hers and away we did go.

The day was real stormy and we were going to drive to the coast to a little place called Capitola by the beach. There was a hotel right on a cliff over-looking the ocean and we had it reserved for a few days and that is where we were headed. We stopped at a fancy restaurant in Palo Alto and by then the wind and rain were strong but we loved it and it made it really cozy. Jean still laughs at my looking for our wedding certificate just in case we would be asked if we were married. I was really naïve.

We arrived at the hotel and found out that we were the only tenants because of the storm so we had the place all to ourselves. The owner asked us to just tell her when we needed our meals and they would be ready and special for the newlyweds. There was a twinkle in her eyes that told her story of when she was our age and now 57 years later I hope that young people will see that same twinkle in our eyes and know yes it can be done.

With the wind and ocean waves pounding the shore it made it so exciting and when we ate our meals we had a window overlooking the beach. We visited the little village and we were so happy to just make up for lost time.

We will never forget those first days of our marriage. We hated to leave but life must go on.

I started working at my old job and I was so surprised that so many people didn't even know we were having a problem in Korea. I felt very out of place when people talked about staying out of other nation's business. I just went along doing my job and getting up to speed. We were settling down to married life and meeting new friends and later on in November our first son, Michael, was born.

We lived in a cute little apartment on the second floor and with our little baby it was just right. In those days we did our own washing of the diapers. No throwaways back then. Just like the stoves. The microwaves were not out yet so Jean cooked our meals the old-fashioned way and we did have some nice mealtimes together. We were too busy to get involved in church work but we always attended Sunday services and special events.

We did a lot of visiting with our family all living close enough so we kept in touch. Almost everyone was having babies so birthdays were becoming more frequent and our life was full of sharing with one another.

We lived in San Francisco for seven years and I was doing fine with my work and we thought we would always be here until we had little Theresa and little Frankie. We always enjoyed the outdoors and we would go visit Jean's sister who moved to Cupertino, a little town 50 miles south from us. Their weather was great all year around and so we always wished that some day we might move down to that area. We started looking for a place a little bigger than we had because with three kids we were getting a little crowded.

My company made it easy for us to decide what to do when they asked me if I would mind moving to Santa Clara, which was real close to Cupertino. What a break! Jean and I never dreamt this would happen but we said yes and this was perfect for our kids with so many outdoor things to do. There were a lot less people living in the area and we could see for miles around under clear blue skies. Our kids loved it and we were still able to visit the family when birthdays came up or to attend special events. During these years the kids would pretty much do the things we told them to do and Jean was at home all the time so she had time with them and a little more room to do it in.

Jean was not driving at that time and all our plans for the future were ahead of us. These years are so special for young couples. Parents are always too busy setting up to do things all the time so kids don't get the attention they need. We put all this in the hands of the Lord and started our new life in Santa Clara.

Chapter Four

Our Years in Santa Clara

Moving to Santa Clara was harder than we expected. We knew it was what we wanted to do but saying good-bye to old friends is never easy. Our families knew it was for the best but still being born and raised in the city meant leaving a lot behind but we managed and started looking ahead to our new life.

The kids were too little to know what was going on and to see us happy was all they had to see. After we moved into our brand new home. They enjoyed playing with their new friends and indoors they had lots of room and we really enjoyed that.

The first few months we did miss the family a lot but then we started getting busy around the house and there was so much to see so we did a little bit at a time and before you knew it we were like we always lived there. Once they started to go to school our life changed because we got involved with their school activities.

Jean helped the students with their reading and I coached basketball and baseball and those were good years.

As our kids began to get into the ten to thirteen years we noticed their peer groups had more influence in their lives than we did. We did not allow our kids to see certain movies while others parents said it was okay and even went to the movies with them. This made it hard to explain to our kids but we managed to hold our ground and with a lot of praying we got through all those years and later our kids told us how good it was to see us hold our ground. We always told them that God did not give us some practice in being parents so we had to learn from our mistakes. Then came those teenage years and that was when TV started to breakdown the families. Parents just gave up and I was so glad we had the Lord on our side because only Jesus could control the evil spirits always seeking to destroy young lives. We still had a lot of heartbreaks as time went on because our kids, being human, fell into bad company and as they got older they would forget the basic truths that we taught them. We were sorry to see that as they began graduating from high school they wanted to live on their own and there was nothing we could do. We now had an empty home and Jean and I sort of felt sad because they were lost and needed our help.

Jean and I began to make our own plan and it was nice to be able to do things without going through our calendars to make sure that we didn't plan something on the same day. It seemed we either had to drive our kids to a game, a show or to a friend's home, etc.

Jean started to feel the need to do something for someone else and a friend told her that the Veterans Hospital in Palo Alto just a half hour away needed someone to work with two Catholic chaplains in visiting the patients and bringing them Communion. I drove her for an appointment and sure enough she was welcomed with open arms and she loved the work.

She started going there one day a week and next thing you know she added two more days and then started to attend classes to become a better volunteer. Now that we had nobody at home we had time to get Jean a driver's license so she could drive herself to the hospital and sure enough we got a car for her and she just loved to finally do things on her own. She never wanted to drive in San Francisco. People get used to taking public transportation and in fact it is better because you don't have to look for a parking place. Here in the country, so to speak, you have to drive a car because some cities have no bus. I loved it when Jean would say, "I will be right back." She would tell me later how much she loved to open up the window and let the wind blow through her hair and listen to the radio. She loved to do the simple things and never wanted much for herself. Little did I dream how her life would change and she would have to depend on someone else for doing everything for her. I say to the young people enjoy every day and know the Lord is with you and loves you. He made you with a purpose in mind so there is a reason for everything that happens to you and we need to let go and let God take over. This life will end for everyone some day and then we will see how it is the beginning of something more beautiful than we could imagine.

Jean always loved doing something for someone else. She had permission to visit anyone she wanted including the lock wards. All the patients (all were men) asked for her and she just listened to what they had to say and would pray with them if they asked her to. I began to attend classes with her when I could so that I could join her one day when I had the time. Little by little we were being drawn closer to the Lord and into this kind of ministry. This also took our mind off the kids and their problems. We worried a lot about them and wondered why this was happening to us. The Lord answered our prayer by sending Jean's brother to visit us with a very timely message. He asked us, "Do we really know Jesus?" We were offended at first because we were doing the best we could to be pleasing to the Lord. What we finally found out was we knew all about Jesus but we did not know Jesus and in a very personal way. We started to attend a prayer meeting that her brother told her about where over one thousand people attended every Friday evening. We were born again! Our life changed and through prayer and by example we drew all our kids back to the Lord and today they tell us that seeing how our lives changed was what turned their life around. I mean not just them but their spouses and all their children. Today when we get together we share the Lord and praise and worship together whenever we can and one thing led to another. We found new friends and attended conventions and seminars. Jean and I found that with the hospital training we had a good base and found it easier to talk to people about their problems and to pray with them whenever they asked God, who is so good, and to let us help Him bring people to Him was so special. We needed no extra work all we needed was to let Him do the work as we brought these special people to him. Jean was kept busy at the hospital and then added some extra volunteer work at our Renewal Center that was set up by the priest who conducted the Friday night prayer meeting.

The center was staffed by volunteers who answered the phones and gave information about our prayer meeting and prayed with the caller if they asked. Many persons dropped in when they heard about our center and it was like our own little church. Our Bishop had 100 % trust in us and we made sure that everyone who came would be active in their own parish and many good things came out of that and we were encouraged to seek the people who dropped out of going to church. Once they discovered the beauty of giving your life to Jesus they came back to their churches and became a busy member of their parish as well. Our kids started to bring their friends to the prayer meetings and to this day they still lead the group that Jean and I started in our parish.

Life was good working for the Lord. We were in our early fifties and full of energy so we were going seven days a week. Jean was blessed with good health and there was no clue that Alzheimer's was going to be developing in her life.

We did a lot of driving around visiting prayer groups and whenever we could help a group leader get started we would do so and in time our bishop appointed me to represent him as a liaison to the Charismatic Renewal. All that meant was that I would report to him whatever we felt he should know so we would always be in the good graces of our church and never stray away from its teaching.

Our biggest thrill was when I was asked to represent our diocese to be with our Pope when he visited San Francisco. That was a beautiful weekend. I was an arm's length away at one time and I still look at that picture I took and can't believe we were there.

We were approaching retirement age and business was slowing down and naturally companies start to cut down on expenses. My boss had two sons coming out of college and I was approaching 62 years of age so I knew I had to take that into consideration. I managed to change to another company but my future was not secure so I mentioned to a friend of mine about my future and he told me that I should look into driving a school bus and retire from my regular job and apply for social security. We had equity built up in our house so all the math added up and that is what I did. I just had to wait a little bit till I turned 62 but in the meantime I was training to be a school bus driver and that was some job. It was like being a teacher in a classroom built on wheels and having your back facing the students all the time. I had to take charge and I guess the kids saw I had a good sense of humor and at the same time I didn't put up with too much of their shenanigans.

We looked at the whole picture and Jean and I decided to move to a small town where we could purchase a nice home for one third less than we would pay in our area. The family saw our need and agreed that was a good plan but the trouble was that with their kids in their teenage years it was not good. They would be leaving their friends and in the town we picked there was nothing to do. We had chosen Turlock, which was 100 miles away and we loved it and the high school was two blocks away. It was a cute little town of 35,000 people. One theater and the kids were quick to point out that they were closing down the bowling alley. We talked it over and saw their point but we decided to move and said we would still see a lot of each other. It was only a two hour ride.

The day came that we sold our home and we were ready to move into that cute corner home with all those tree lined streets and real country.

Chapter Five

Living in Turlock

After 41 years in Santa Clara it was not easy packing up and leaving our old home. This is where our kids grew up. We had a lot of heartbreak as well as real happy times while living on Las Palmas Drive. The two story yellow house had started as a three bedroom two bath home and we added three more bedrooms and one more bathroom as the kids got older and needed more space. Jean was the last to leave and she took her time sweeping out the house just as if she was sweeping out all the memories.

Finally we all piled into our cars and followed the big moving van on to Turlock. We unloaded and ordered some pizza and drinks and all sat in the kitchen and realized that as soon as we finished our family would leave us and head back to Santa Clara without us. That was the hard part but we had talked all this over and it was the best way for us to go. That was a lot of trauma for Jean and I knew she was holding back tears for a few days. Moments like these cause the start of Alzheimer's in some cases and later I felt this may have been the time Jean began to be affected. We had no friends so it was like we had gone camping all by ourselves and with no one around to go to in time of need. We planned on buying appliances and so we had coolers and a camping stove to get along with and it was fun to rough it out till we furnished the kitchen and laundry room.

All that stuff was over 15 years old so we left it behind to make it more attractive to sell the home.

I had been hired as a bus driver for the Turlock School District so I reported bright and early the next morning and here we were business as usual. Two hours in the morning and two in the afternoon. Jean got used to the new house and she was kept busy putting things away and planning get a garden going. We had a lot of fun getting used to things and it wasn't long before we were asked to join the various church organizations.

The church was two blocks away and we also were asked to join the Stockton Laison's group. We knew some of the people from previous meetings we attended when we met with all eight Northern California Charismatic laisons as we planned state-wide events. It was good that we were still involved in the group. The churches in the valley were smaller and more friendly and the work was all the same so we got right in on what we had been doing in Santa Clara. The students were also different in ways hard to describe. They were calmer and very polite. They showed no interest in going to the Bay area. They would rather go fishing boating or skiing and hiking. All the things our grand kids never wanted to do. We did our share of most of those things when we took time off for ourselves. We could now say we loved living out here. We never missed a birthday or special family event and we were feeling right at home. We had all the time in the world to get used to our new surroundings and get to know all these new friends.

I was doing my bus driving thing and Jean filled in her time at the hospital and rest homes and she loved it. Our church asked Jean to also visit some people in their homes and she took that on so I could see she was really enjoying going from one place to another. I kept on driving the kids to school for about

7 years and finally we decided to fully retire and I would join Jean and start doing things together as we liked to do.

Our visits to the homes was still something we did on our own but the hospital and rest homes we did together and later we expanded our knowledge in visiting patients by taking courses in spiritual care sponsored by the hospital. This was real helpful because more and more people from all over the world were moving into town and we had to know their culture so we did not offend them as we tried to make them feel comfortable. This was so helpful as we worked some days in the emergency section and we met the whole family all at once and they wanted to know everything as soon as possible. We were able to calm them down and take away their fears and then all went smoothly from then until the doctor arrived. The Lord led us even further into this ministry by getting us into Hospice work. This is dealing with a patient who is terminally ill. We volunteered to get into Hospice care and attended a forty hour course to be certified. This is just the beginning. There is a lot of hands on experience we get by working with the patients, doctors, nurses and family. Jean loved the work and so did I.

Time went by and our family was growing up and we saw them a lot on week ends and once in awhile they would come and stay with us for a couple of days. We always loved volunteering because we could do it on our own time and the work was rewarding. Of course no pay but in the end we get a big bonus. We always kidded about us always doing some thing with our spare time. What is spare time? We thought we had some until we attended a home-owners meeting. The guest speaker was a man in charge of a new group being formed by the Turlock Police Department. This group would be known as Volunteers in Patrol. Their duty was to patrol the city in regular police cruisers and report any problems needing police attention. Jean was real excited about it but I felt reluctant in getting involved but I just felt she was so wanting to do it so we signed up and it was a real good choice. We trained at the police station for a six month period two nights a week and we were taught how to use the radio and deal with the traffic control situations and all about police work. We wore uniforms and seeing the smile on Jean's face on graduation night made me so proud of her. She had a badge and her own equipment and she was ready to go and off we went. Our granddaughter was training to be a police officer herself and she was thrilled to know what we were doing. One day she came to visit us and we arranged for her to go out with a K-9 car as a guest and we went out in our own cruiser. Two hours later we were called to direct traffic at an intersection accident and here was Jean our granddaughter and me directing traffic. That was a sight to see. All three together smiling at each other and wondering is this for real?

In all the things we did there were a lot of beautiful things that happened and we could write about so many ways the Lord used us but this is about Jean who gave of her time and asked for no more than to please God and family. As we started to pull back as her condition worsened I just wanted to bring out the pure joy a simple life could bring to others when it is done in the spirit of giving and the Lord working through each one of us. If we let Him!

Chapter Six

The Challenge of Alzheimer's Disease

Up till now I've covered 57 years of marriage to the most beautiful woman I have ever met. I see the beauty of God's design in her. She radiates the love of Jesus and with her smile she brings out the best in people. Of course I have seen her when she was very angry when I did some thing very wrong and also very disappointed in me when I ignored the signs telling me to use caution instead of just plunging ahead and then it was too late to change. But then I saw how she was always willing to reach out to me and forgive me and put everything behind us and go for a fresh start. She always let me have all the credit when things went right and she was always that way with people. She always let others take the bows and she enjoyed doing that. This is why it hurt so much to see her get Alzheimer's instead of having good health and look ahead at some more good years. Alzheimer's robs people of their memories and the ability to do things. I felt so bad when I had to tell Jean that I would have to drive her from now on. She loved her freedom when she hopped into her car and went shopping. She knew it was not possible to learn how to do things all over again. Alzheimer's patients cannot be taught to do things. She could no longer type on her computer and she would always get lost when she would leave the house not to mention losing her car in parking lots. She was so cute when she would call me on the cell phone and ask for help.

One time she called me to find out when I was going to pick her up and did not remember if she took her car. I had to tell the manager of the store to see if he could see her car and sure enough he did and Jean drove home. The danger in driving is that with Alzheimer's one could get into a serious accident and it would be our fault not to mention some one could get killed. That is why the Department of Motor vehicles wants to have you stop driving once you are diagnosed with Alzheimer's.

Jean was good about giving it all up. I felt bad because I wanted to give her so many things to make up for times she had to do without. I should know better. She didn't keep score and wait to get even. She was content and that was why I always felt so blest when she would thank me for buying her dinner. Imaging after 57 years she thanked me for that. I should be thanking her for putting up with me. I tell all the young couples that ask me for advice to always tell your partner you love them and treasure every moment you share. With kids and the job and other things that keep you busy it's so important to have a time for just the two of you and hear a thank you. One time Jean left me a note of one word in letters about three inches and just the word yes.

When we walked we always held hands. She was a great hand holder and I could feel her squeeze my hand as she would tell me she was having such a good time. Those are great moments and good to recall when I need a boost. My heart was broken when she could no longer speak and tell me lots of little things that were so important to her. Then when I sometimes got preoccupied she would stop and smile and say, "You're not listening." Then she would tell me about the language of the heart. Always listen to my heart she would say. "You won't know a person if you don't know their heart."

Again I say to young couples, "Learn to listen. It may not be important to you but one day you will hear your loved one tell you that you listen to others much more than you. Then you will know what I mean." I mentioned before that Jean would speak with her eyes and hand motion but I longed to hear her voice again. When I am alone I could hear her voice in my heart. I can't say enough, "Treasure all those moments," they are precious.

From 2004 we had lots of fun and did the best we could. She knew she had my love and so when she needed my help I was there and she let me take over. I was committed to be with her every minute so if she got into trouble I could find a way out of a bad situation.

We sure came up with different types of problems but we laughed through them all and I always knew how much she appreciated my trying to do something for her. Sometimes we had to come home early because she was having trouble but she saw I was not disappointed and her love and my love took care of the rest. We actually felt stronger in our love and started out each day ready to face another challenge. The support group we attended was so important because we made real good friends and we were able to grow and face things together. Every week we could share about what we had problems with and others could tell us what worked for them. Sometimes that was what we needed to do and if it didn't work at least we were able to get it off our chest and feel that we were not alone in our fight against Alzheimer's Disease. When we stopped volunteering and lost the friendship from the people we saw all the time, the caregivers we met were much closer to us then even members of our family. No one knows what we face unless they too have someone they are taking care of. Even then no two cases are the same. The part we all shared was the knowledge we were seeking about this disease and what we could do to help one another to cope. The fact that there is no end to our days and our loved ones have a new challenge daily is why meeting every week with others is so important.

I always felt blessed that Jean knew who I was. I heard others tell how they no longer were known to the patient. I felt so sad but at the same time I was glad for them that they were not alone and were supported when they needed to be listened to.

When the time came to place our loved one in long term care it was a task that you needed help with.

Where do you go? How do you tell your loved one that you no longer could take care of them at home? We forget how many times we said it would never happen. Then the time comes when your doctor tells you that you are going to get sick yourself and then who will take over. Usually no one will do what you did. You have to decide what is good for all.

The Lord helped me out when my time came. Jean was so badly injured with a fall in our bathroom that she was taken to a hospital. During her stay our doctor was able to tell Jean how much she would benefit at a long term care facility and I would be able to see her as much as I could. Of course she thought she would come home when she got better but then tomorrow is another day.

She stayed 18 months and I can't feel I let her down. We were blessed that we found an opening at a rest home that we volunteered at for 17 years and knowing the people was such a good thing. Jean felt comfortable from the start and they all loved her and treated her with much loving tender care. We were together every day. I would come in at 11:30 and leave after dinner. Being home alone was tough and I sure missed her but after a few months I realized how much sleep I was not able to get by getting up at all hours when Jean was home. The doctor was right. My health got better and I was committed to being with Jean. She was home to me. I wanted to be there. Days off were not an option. She waited for me at the same time every day and could light up the world with the smile she gave me when she first spotted me and we went from there. We had a lot of things to do with the activities planned for the patients thanks to Glady and her group of helpers who kept everyone on their toes and morale at a constant high. The nurses all came running to Jean when she asked for help so I was very satisfied that she was being taken care of. Of course Alzheimer's keeps taking its toll and Jean developed problems in digesting and chewing her food so they put her on pureed food. It didn't look too good on a plate but it did the job and Jean never complained. Then I was told that her system was breaking down and to expect the worse in the near future. There is no good way to present this situation because we all could suggest some thing that may work. Maybe someday we can cure Alzheimer's Disease but for now we can only pray. Jean still had her best smile on every moment of the day. I know she was already in Heaven and just waiting for her call. Our daughter and son came to see her on the week-end of President's day and we had a great visit. Jean was happy and when we said our good-byes it seemed that my Jean was ready.

I was home around 8:30 and was recalling how good the day was and glad Theresa and Frank came because they too felt the time had come. The phone call came at 10:10 p.m. and the nurse told me Jean had passed away. It hurt so bad. I was silent for a while and I asked how much time I had before the funeral people would come and she said two hours. So I hurried up and was at her side and I had the most beautiful two hours all alone with her holding her hand and seeing her so at peace. I remember telling Jean to make sure Jesus doesn't forget me and she had smiled as if to say I did already and I know she is so happy waiting for me and all our family. We all know that is our destiny and as St. Paul says in his letter to the Corinthians. "Eye has not seen, ear has not heard, nor has it so much as dawned on man what God has prepared for those who love Him."